Note to reader:

The reader assumes all responsibilities with regard to use or sharing of any and all information in this booklet. The use of force outside the situation of self-defense is unlawful and must be avoided! Please consult local laws re: permissible use of force.

The pictures depicted in this body of work are not meant to teach actual techniques. I have used hypothetical scenarios to help convey the possibilities for the use of your natural and improvised weapons.

DEDICATED TO MY MOTHER RUTH AND MY MELISSA,
THEY INSPIRE ME TO DREAM AND TO LOVE WITH ALL MY HEART!

Finger break, bite.
Use anything
available to escape.

Introduction

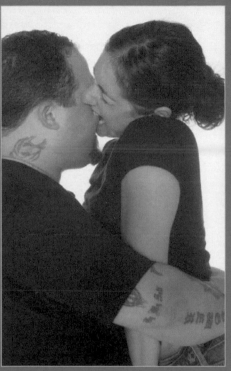

BAD THINGS HAPPEN TO GOOD PEOPLE EVERYDAY.

How many stories have you heard of women screaming for help and no one coming in the middle of the day, even at a busy park or office building? They were on their own!

My intention with this information is to prepare women with ideas that will help them deal with life threatening situations. Forget about all the people who've said you're too weak and small; the **will to survive** must be the driving force fueling your escape. Dig down deep, past the fear and find your survival state of mind, a mindset of, I'm going to get through this, nothing and no one is going to prevent me from saving my life! **Let fear make you run, let fear make you fight, never, never let fear keep you standing still.** Right here, right now, Body, Mind and Spirit, all focused on your survival. If you only take one thing from this book, let it be this: you don't have to be a statistic with no control over your situation; you can take action to save your life or someone else's.

I've put together some basic information every woman should know. It doesn't rely on strength or size. It relies on strategy and preparation, some attention to detail and some basic practice. Strength can be overcome with planning and practice. With a plan of action you can stay one step ahead of the bad guy (or bad situation) and turn that fear energy of a life threatening situation into get moving energy and save your life.

Note: Physical attacks or attempts at abduction require an immediate physical response, be it fighting back, drawing attention by yelling and screaming, running away or even possibly blowing a whistle, anything that will give you the opportunity to escape.

The body, being the awesome machine that it is, comes with its own arsenal of natural tools (weapons). I will describe them. Refer back to the Weapons chapter from time to time to refresh your memory of them. Your ability to recall and apply these ideas will depend directly on your effort to know them. Practice is the only way to increase your chances of retaining the information and your ability to apply it.

Think about each defense and how you might put it into use, along with the ideas that I've included. **Remember there are no rules when saving your life,** there are predators who roam the streets who will not think twice about ruining a life for the gain of a few bucks or to fulfill a sick desire.

Note: It's important that you remember your first line of defense, escape (avoidance), which you must consider before engaging a person in any physical confrontation. If you can leave the area safely without incident, you must. Use the system whenever possible; involve the authorities sooner than later when your safety is in question.

I've protected people, money and property for many years and one thing holds true. Planning and practice have been my most valuable assets with regard to the unforeseen situations that arise during a normal day's business.

This is about self-defense but more specifically, survival defense, about preparing for life's unexpected life-threatening situations and the bad guys that may come with them.

Instead of thinking, "Oh God, what do I do now?" you will be aware of your choices and have a head start in a situation with little or no time to think.

I repeat your ability to recall and apply these ideas will depend directly on your effort to know them. Skill levels acquired in any defense or survival training are achieved with practice. Study them, refer back to them, and know them! In my experience with self-defense training, it has become very clear to me that techniques are very difficult to learn from a book. A book can't tell you to shift your weight here and there at the very moment you're doing it wrong; it can't reposition your body for you. This information is not only for women. It's for all the people who know that safety is a primary function of life and still do nothing about it. Everyone hears that they must exercise and eat right and they still don't. Well not exercising and not eating right will definitely catch up to you eventually.

A life-threatening situation can happen at anytime, even while you're reading this guide. Are you ready? Who are you going to blame when you're not prepared? Use the information in this guide as your first step to taking responsibility for your own safety. Then take the next step and get some training.

Elbow strike.

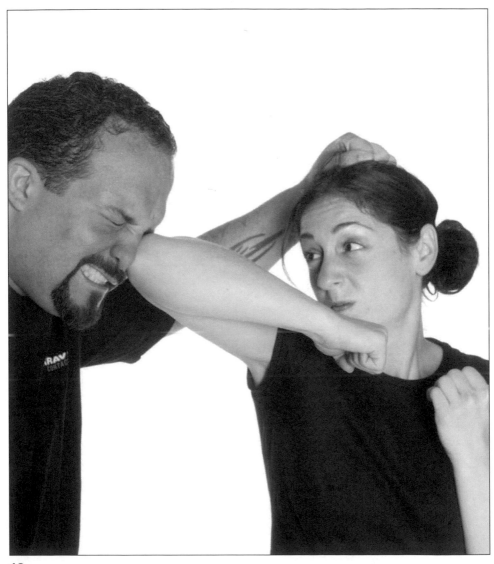

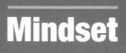

Mindset

Your state of mind

The right state of mind starts with awareness. It is common to feel panic and anxiety in an uncertain situation, especially a life-threatening emergency such as a fire or an attack. Knowledge and forethought will help with the confusion of an unexpected occurrence.

One specific thing I'd like to call attention to is your state of mind during these situations. Through experience and conversation I have found that people respond sooner when helping or protecting another individual, especially a child or loved one. The fight or flight response seems to kick in quicker when an individual sees that danger is imminent for child, loved one or friend. How many stories have you heard where a person says "I saw the fire or the man came out of no where and I just froze"? Where, on the other hand, you hear that a five foot one hundred pound woman defends her family against a much larger attacker or had carried someone twice her size to safety. These thoughts of protecting another person can be a great tool in helping to keep you focused on the situation at hand. Thinking of your loved ones will help you to get going and keep you moving. Protect your space: be aware of who's in it and what they are doing. Everyone is subject to scrutiny of agenda when it comes to your personal space. Always remember, getting out of harm's way is our ultimate goal. Excessive force such as continuing to injure an attacker that is already down is against the law. Stay focused on your goal; to escape safely with little or no injury.

Having a plan of action and practicing the movements that you might employ will help with the shock of a life-threatening event. Preparation is wasted without being aware of your environment. The first line of defense is awareness so you can avoid potential dangers.

Be aware of distraction tactics: asking for the time, change or directions. It's okay to be nice; it's dangerous to be too comfortable. People with bad intentions prey on the kindness of people they can get close to.

As soon as you notice a person who is getting close, ask yourself, "What's up with this person? And why is this person in my personal space without reason or invitation?" Your personal space is the distance you can reach with any part of your body in a 360 degree radius. Of course your environment may change this, as in being in a small area such as an elevator or a crowded public space. In these situations you must be weary of any and all contact. Note: a simple bump could be a distraction for a pick pocket, or creepy guy trying to get a cheap thrill on a crowded bus or train.

Peripheral vision – Along with awareness a person's primary line of defense is vision. If you can see a potential danger, the surprise factor is decreased (but not totally gone since you don't know the bad guy's intentions). You can initiate a protective course of action, be it getting the attention of others, changing direction and putting space in between you and the person. Or if time or space does not permit those actions prepare to physically defend yourself.

Here's an exercise:

While looking forward I would like you to explore your true range of vision. You can see (without turning your head or with the slightest turn), a lot more than what's just in front of you. With practice you will be able to get a full frontal view, side view and a fraction of what's just slightly behind you without moving your head. Getting comfortable with this natural ability will increase your chances of avoiding a situation.

Please note: One big aggressive step from two adults standing ten feet apart will put them in striking distance of each other.

When walking, one must scan their immediate area every few blocks or so, especially heading home from local stores. Complacency sets in when you're close to home. Notice people who are acting strangely, wearing odd attire for weather requirements, such as a hooded jacket when it's warm, hands hidden behind clothing or newspaper and people intentionally avoiding eye contact.

Awareness Zone 20ft – When a person comes into the awareness zone, what are they doing? Are they just walking by, have they looked at you? Take notice of the person's demeanor; get an idea of their mood from their facial expressions. Is their pace and stride casual or purposeful, or is it hesitant, with odd pauses? This is your first opportunity to assess someone's intentions as they are about to enter your personal space. At this distance you should have noticed any people approaching you, their appearance, attire and demeanor.

Caution zone 10-20ft – As a person crosses into this space you must survey their intentions. Are they paying attention to you? Take notice of the person's attire. Don't be fooled by a clean cut appearance, but definitely trust in the obvious. More often than not bad guys dress the part: wearing dark clothes and hoods to try and hide their faces and physical features, wearing multiple layers of clothing so they can change their appearance quickly. Once again access the person's body language; and ask yourself, "Do I feel comfortable?"

Danger Zone from your body to 10ft around you – Has that little voice in your head been shouting at you that something doesn't feel right? At this point you can change direction if you feel the situation isn't right. You can attract attention verbally or by blowing a whistle; you can advise this person or persons that you are aware and that you don't want them to come any closer. You can get your cell phone ready to call for help (**911 should be preprogrammed in your cell phone for one button operation**). Jump right into your primary defense actions: shouting, raising your opened hands in a stop fashion and say sternly "**STOP**, do not come any closer". If at this time, none of these actions has deterred the person's course of action or direction, you must leave the area if you can do so safely (call 911), try to get something in between you and the person; a car, other people anything available and be ready to defend yourself.

Call the authorities and report the incident. Give a description of the perpetrator as soon as possible. This will flood the area with law enforcement and raise the chances of catching the perpetrator. Believe it or not criminals often commit crimes very close to home. Remember not reporting the incident will leave a criminal out on the streets to do it again.

Note: Assailants and robbers generally look for easy prey, marks or targets. Attitude with regard to your facial expression and body language, such as walking tall and taking assertive strides will help to deter either. Sluggish appearance or looking tired and distracted will signal an assailant that you are unaware and probably not prepared to defend yourself against his agenda (talking on a cell phone, listening to an ipod or carrying too many bags).

Scenario: Should someone make a verbal advance to you. Try to be polite with a nod or a thank you. Stay alert and keep moving. As much as I want you to be strong and assertive, being too aggressive can trigger a negative response from a potential perpetrator. As I've said before being nice is ok, being too comfortable may be dangerous, just as well, being too aggressive (mean) can possibly spark a situation that could have been avoided.

Some women will feel that they're too weak to defend themselves against a larger or stronger adversary. While the attacker may believe that you will not be prepared for a fight, this is life or death, and you're going to give it everything you've got. You have prepared mentally and practiced physically so that your options are fresh in your mind. You will not be defending against the might or size of an attacker; you will be attacking his/ her weakest points (refer to Primary Targets Section). You are not fighting a 250lb man; you will be fighting two eyes, a throat, a nose, a jaw, a groin, fingers, any and all targets available to you so that you can escape. You must objectify your attacker....think of him as body parts....for all you know he's all bark. One thing for sure is, you're prepared to bite, punch, kick, tear, slap, poke and stay focused on your goal to escape safely, period!

Physical attack requires a physical response. The only defensive actions to invest energy in are to flee or block a weapon. All other defensive actions do nothing to stop a physical attack. You must disable the perpetrator's ability to continue his actions.

REMEMBER, ESCAPING SAFELY IS THE PRIMARY GOAL ALTHOUGH IT MAY BE A LARGE INCONVENIENCE TO REPLACE VALUABLES LOST IN A ROBBERY, IT IS NO COMPARISON TO INJURY OR LOSS OF LIFE.

With regard to weapons of the body or any everyday item used as a weapon, there are no rules for application. Fighting off an attack will be chaos; your thoughts will be all over the place as well as your emotions. An attacker may not expose the vital areas that you are trying to focus on, so you will attack any part of his body that is exposed until you feel you have the opportunity to attempt an escape.

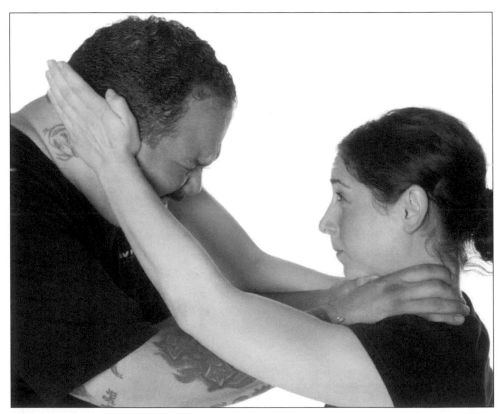

Weapons

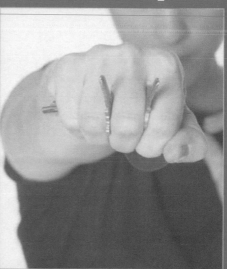

Reviewing this guide from time to time will keep the choices you have available to you fresh in your mind, along with the three primary areas for your offensive defense the **face, throat and groin**. You may have been pushed to the ground. You may not be facing your attacker. **Do something**, anything, to get you free and out of there. Overwhelm your attacker by any means: scream, slap, poke, kick, shout, gouge, stomp, knee, elbow, head butt. Use any item available to you; a comb, brush, lipstick case, shoe (heel), belt buckle, ear ring, ear tear, finger break, throat chop, punch, bite, kick. You get the idea. **Distract, disable and escape.**

Natural defenses of the body

These defenses that I will list for you have no precedent over one another. Try the ones that you feel most comfortable with and keep going until you're able to flee safely. Later I will describe the primary attack areas that give you the most advantage and quickest possibility for escape. **If the perpetrator can't see you, breathe well or move well, he will not be able to continue his actions. REMEMBER, NEVER GIVE UP!**

A Ready Stance sends a clear message that you are ready and pre- pared to respond to the situation, but still allows for verbal defusing. Hands up and open in a stop position, you're repeating clearly that you do not want any trouble, loudly and assertively, even if you don't feel that way inside, it doesn't matter. If you can leave the area safely, do so. Defend offensively if attacked so that you can achieve your ultimate goal of escaping from the attack area. I also would like to make it clear that there is nothing lost if you have misjudged a person's intentions. If you have blown your whistle and shouted for the person to stand back and the person seems surprised at your actions, all you have to say is, "sorry my mistake" and go about you business. Don't let your guard down. Who knows, maybe you judged right and changed what was really about to happen.

Ready stance.

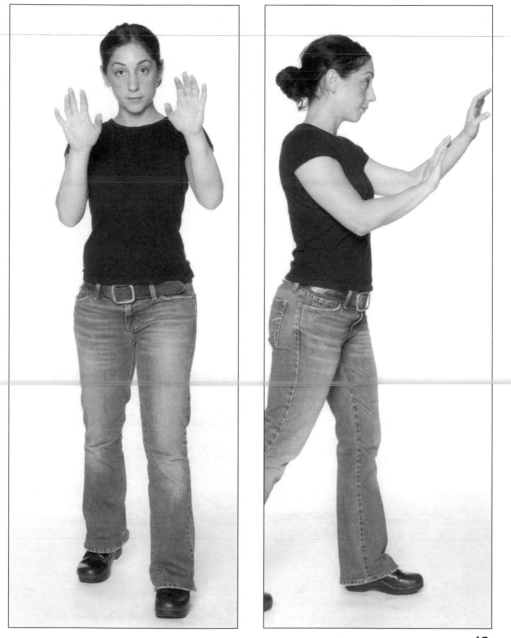

Shouting: A commanding "stop" or "stand back" may be all that's required to alert a person that you're aware of their presence and that you are uncomfortable and serious. For this situation I recommend the purchase of a standard police whistle. It will provide a loud way of getting attention and help you to conserve energy and can also help with other potentially dangerous situations.

Legs and feet: Your legs and feet are the longest and strongest amongst your arsenal of natural body weapons. They will keep an attacker at the furthest distance from your body and will cause damage. Also remember that if you're shoved to the ground you must try to keep your legs and feet in between you and an attacker. If he is still trying to approach you make him pay with the best kicks and stomps you can put together. Do whatever you must to get back on your feet and out of there!

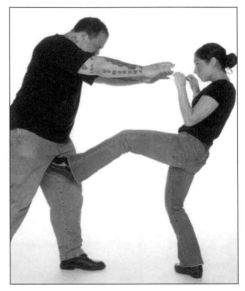

Hands: Keeping your hands up and open in front of you will give you opportunities to strike an attacker as well as giving you some defensive coverage. You will also be able to grab and hold a hand that may have a weapon in it and keep it away from your body.

Note: Keeping your hands open maximizes their use. Make a fist only when you need one!

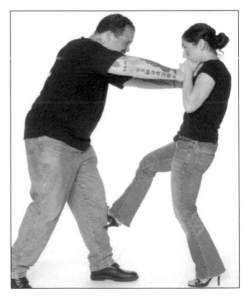

Kicks keep your attacker
at a distance.
Top left, Groin kick
Bottom left, Shin kick with
heel (can be to knee)
This page, Groin kick

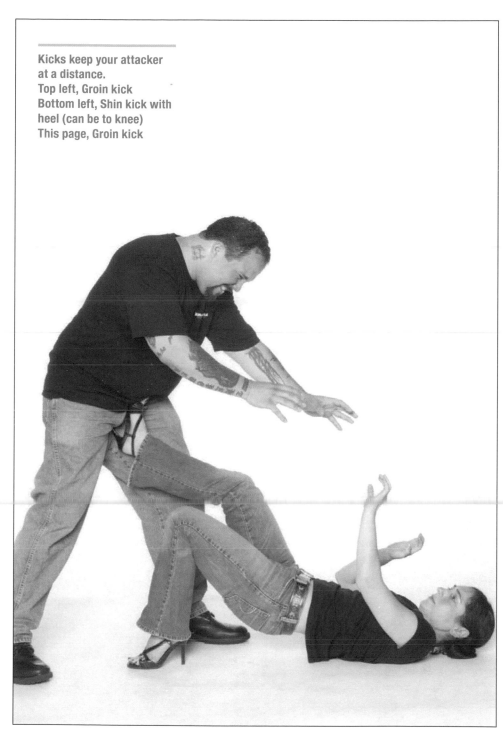

Punches: Using the big knuckles to make impact, punch towards the face, throat, and groin area.

Fingers: poking at the eyes, using a single finger or multiple fingers. This defense will seem hard for some people to imagine doing. This may be your only way of escaping without help from another person or the police? Full penetration of the eye with the finger is not necessary. A firm poke will close the perpetrator's eyes momentarily to allow for other offensive strikes.

Chops: Using the outer ridge of the palm (pinky side of the hand) to attack the face, throat and groin

Palm Strike: A very powerful strike using the base of the palm with an open forward facing hand to strike.

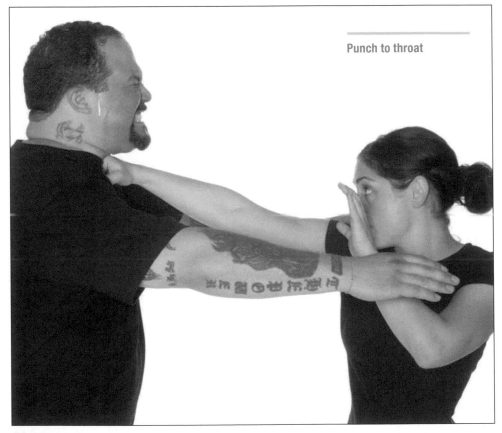

Punch to throat

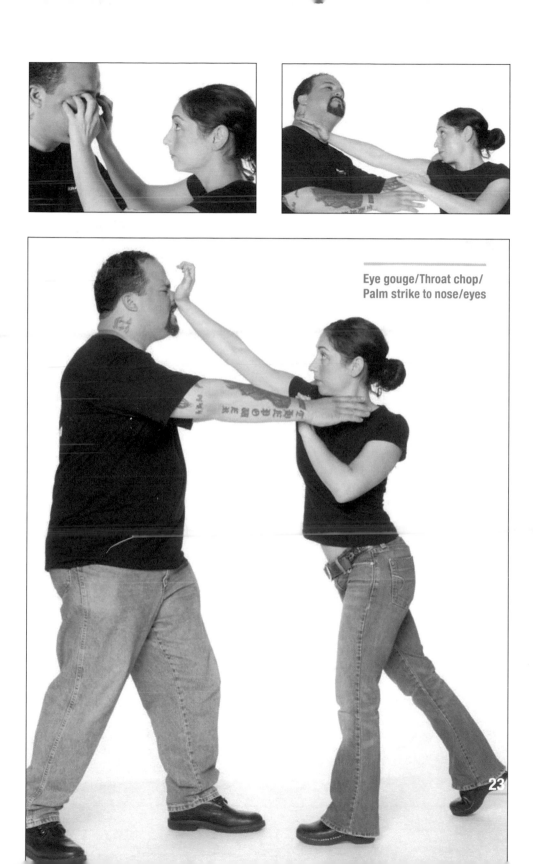

**Eye gouge/Throat chop/
Palm strike to nose/eyes**

**Knee strike to face
(pull your attacker down)**

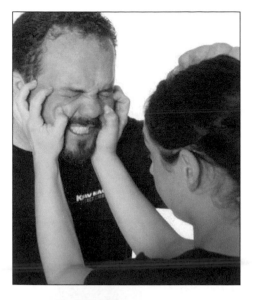

Hair pulling: A simple way to cause damage and possibly control an attacker so that you may employ additional strikes to primary areas

Scratching/ Gouging: at any part of the body. This will cause pain and damage. It may also be a way of identifying an attacker at a later time. DNA from the skin under fingernails can be used to identify an attacker with a previous record, which may include a DNA sample.

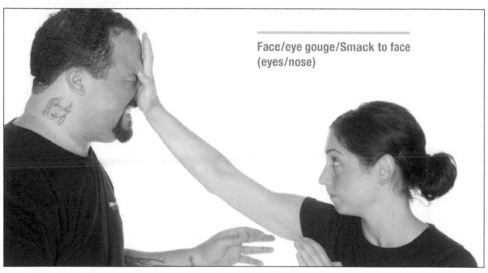

Face/eye gouge/Smack to face (eyes/nose)

Note: Never turn your back on an attacker until you have enough distance to run away safely. Keep trying to get attention with shouts, a whistle, banging on cars to set off alarms, anything that will alert people that something is wrong.

Slapping: A quick movement that can be shocking and painful, target the eyes, nose, ears and groin.

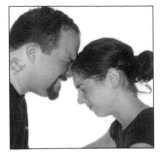

Head: Your head comes into play if an attacker is very close, using your upper forehead along the hair line or the back of your head to strike the facial area of an attacker

Note: Try to always keep your eyes open.

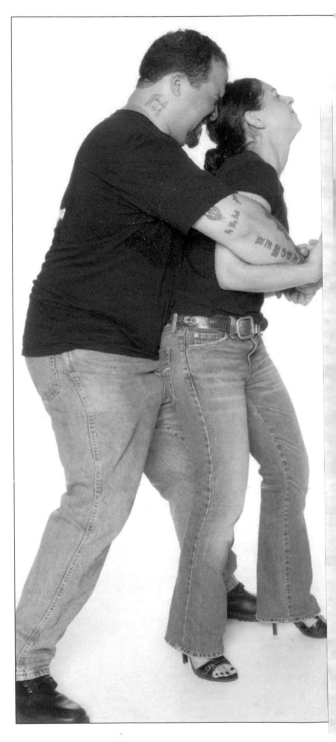

Hammer Fist: A fist used for pounding using a motion that a hammer would make. This is a very strong movement especially for those who don't think they can throw a solid punch. Strike the face, throat and groin area first whenever possible. Attacking any part of the body if those targets are not available may open an opportunity for strikes to those areas. Remember all you want is time to escape. Using both hands in conjunction with some elbows, knees and kicks will raise your chances for the opportunity to escape safely.

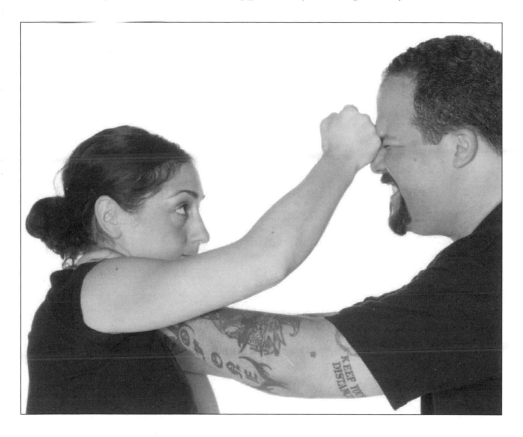

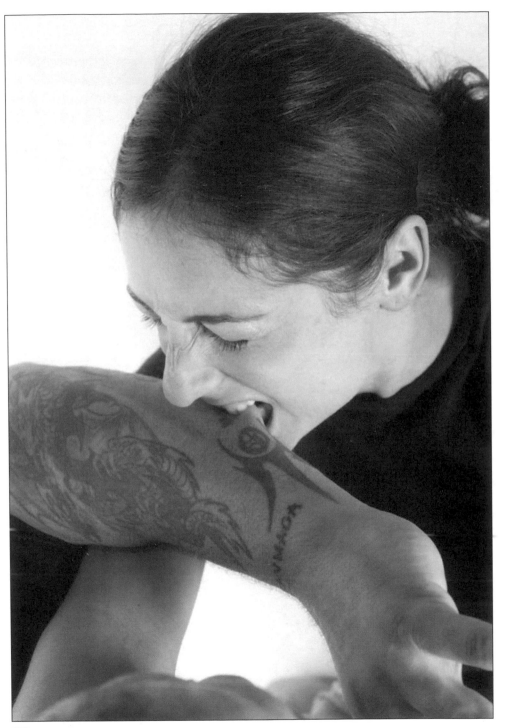

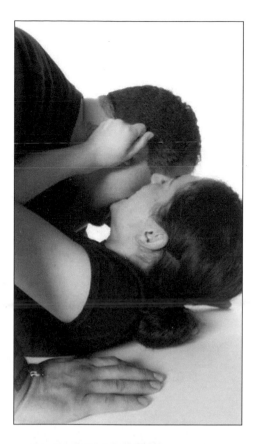

Biting: bite, bite and bite any part, anywhere, this will get a reaction and cause pain that will change an attacker's priorities quickly.

Spitting: towards the eyes or mouth may seem out of sorts for some, but will get a reaction from most if not all. Two seconds may be all the distraction time you need to get a kick to groin or strike to the face and give you the opportunity to get out of there.

Note: Causing pain to an attacker may not be possible due to drugs, alcohol or a mental disorder. You must affect a perpetrator's vision, breathing or movement in some way, so you can stop their attack and escape safely.

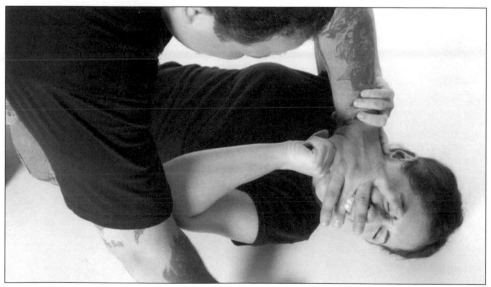

Elbows and Knees: These particular parts of the body are awesome when it comes to offense because they are hard as hell and cause lots of damage with impact or even glancing blows.

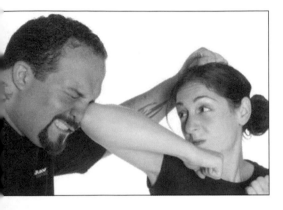

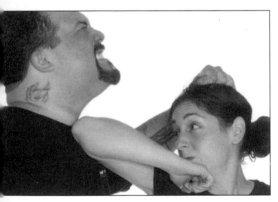

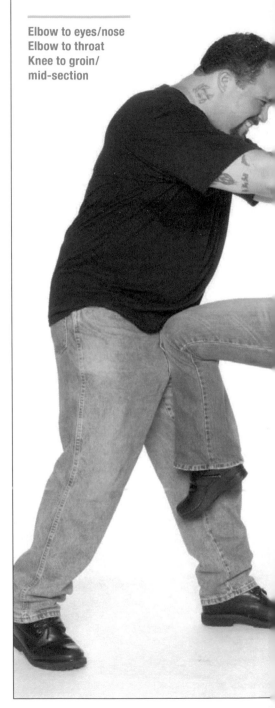

Elbow to eyes/nose
Elbow to throat
Knee to groin/
mid-section

Remember, your goal is distraction by means of pain and or damage which will interrupt or cease an attacker's ability to continue his actions. You must flee the area as soon as physically possible and notify the authorities.

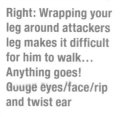

Right: Wrapping your leg around attackers leg makes it difficult for him to walk... Anything goes! Gouge eyes/face/rip and twist ear

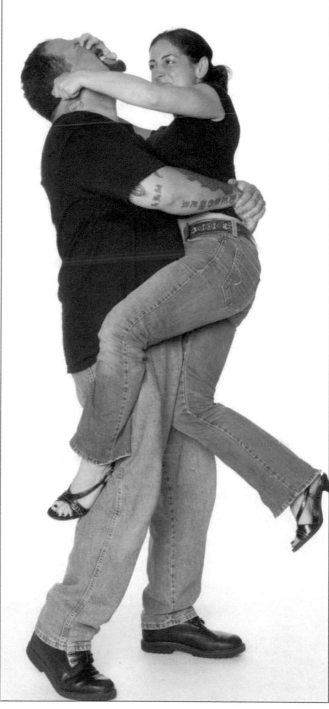

Everyday items that can be used to stop an attacker:

Keys: First and foremost, your keys are an excellent tool that can be used to help you in several different ways. Have them ready in hand, key ready to go. They can be thrown like a projectile at the face as a distraction so you might flee the situation, or set up for a more aggressive offensive defense such as a kick, knee or punch. Your keys can also be wedged between your fingers; (car key, or any large key), so that you can add to the effectiveness of your punches. In a situation where keys are on a long chain they can be used to keep an assailant at a safe distance by swinging the keys aggressively. Fumbling with keys outside your home or vehicle is a perfect opportunity for a perpetrator to get the jump on you.

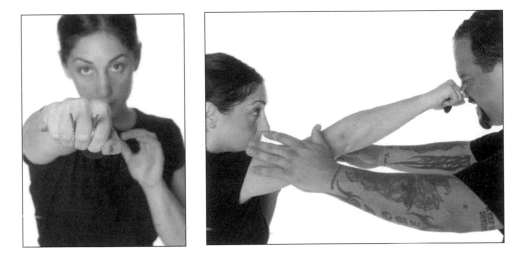

Keys wedged in between fingers while punching

Belt: Your belt can be pulled off and swung at an attacker using the belt buckle to strike. It can also be used to keep an attacker from getting any closer.

Cosmetic cases: These items can be used to strike an assailant and can also be thrown at an attacker. Also included are: brushes, combs, nail file, hair clip, eye wear, lipstick case, eye liner pencil, mascara case.

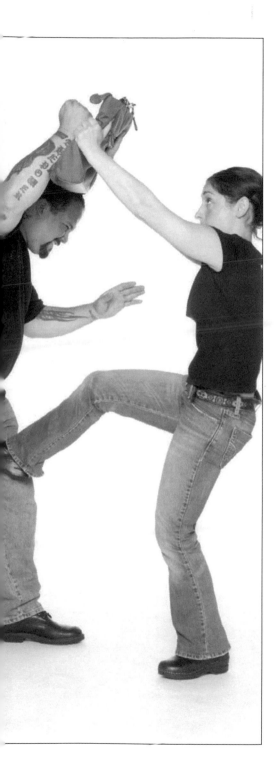

Bag or Briefcase: Anything that you might be carrying, a purse, handbag or shopping bag can be used to shield yourself or strike an assailant.

Umbrella: stabbing and shielding.

Laptop: can be used as a shield and to strike an attacker.

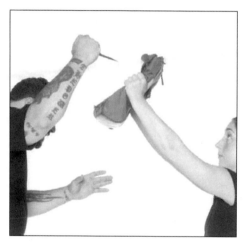

Remember, there are no rules! You must utilize any and all options when it comes to getting an opportunity to escape from an attack or an attempt to move you to a second location.

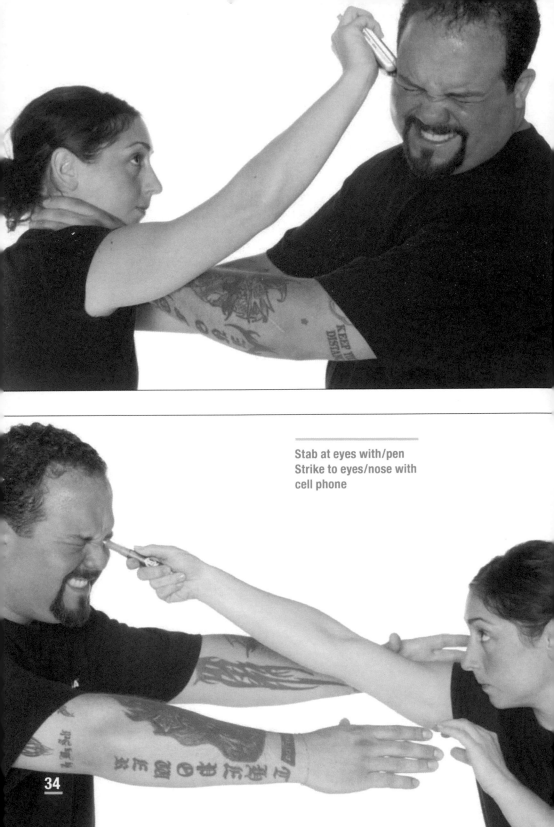

Stab at eyes with/pen
Strike to eyes/nose with
cell phone

Writing Instrument: stabbing; jotting down the details of an incident and identifying features of an attacker; ex: license plate number, make and model of vehicle, facial features, color of hair, color of eyes.

Book: use the corners to strike, use the book to shield against a strike or weapon.

Rolled up Newspaper or Magazine: use to strike, poke, or shield.

Bag of Groceries: throw contents of bag.

Cell phone: strike using phone.

Eyeglasses: can be used to stab at the eyes.

Beverage: can be thrown at assailants face, hot beverage even better can be thrown at the assailants face to cause distraction, (hot beverage will do great in this scenario).

There are no rules! You must utilize any and all options when trying to create an opportunity to escape an attack or attempt at abduction.

Understand: Either you do something when physically attacked or the perpetrator will do whatever he wants. Even if you comply, serious injury and the possibility of death still remain.

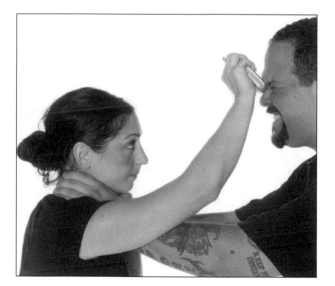

If face is in range strike quickly with cell phone or any object...you must roopond quickly to being choked! You only have a few seconds!

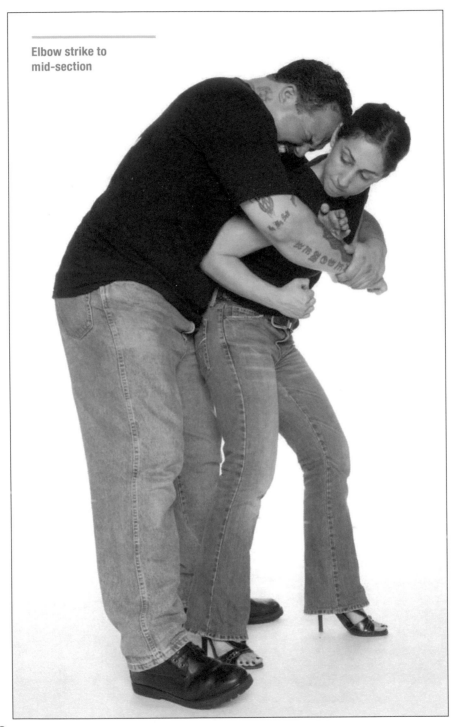

Targets

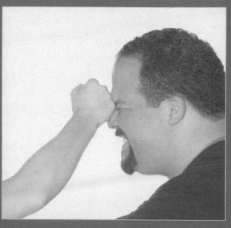

Face
Throat
Groin
Anywhere Anyhow
escape

In this section I will cover the primary areas your offense should be directed to. The **face** (eyes, nose and jaw line), **throat** and **groin**; any of these areas when struck will get you a response. Of course, you will want to attack these areas with a strong sense of purpose because you may be limited to only a few seconds. As the saying goes, sometimes the best defense is a good offense. In fact with regard to self-defense the only defense is offense. (**You must be proactive, mentally and physically. Planning is offense. Practicing is offense. Running is offense. Remember you're using offense for defensive purposes**).

The pain/response induced by attacking these areas will allow for a secondary attack if needed, or may be enough to deter an attacker. The only thing you focus on is going through, over or around the assailant as quickly and effectively as possible to achieve your main goal of getting to safety.

Area / Type of attack (standing or on the ground)

Face: fingers to the eyes, hands, fists, biting, kicking, elbows, head butt (using the crown of the head, just above the forehead to strike), smack, finger rake, hand chop to bridge of nose, flat palm to bridge of nose or eye ridge, nails, or any defense tool you might have a chance to implement.

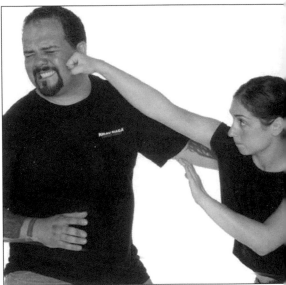

Throat: chops, punches, pinching, finger jab, elbows, biting, kicking, knees, or any defense tool you might have a chance to implement.

Kicking to the throat from the ground... especially effective with heeled shoes

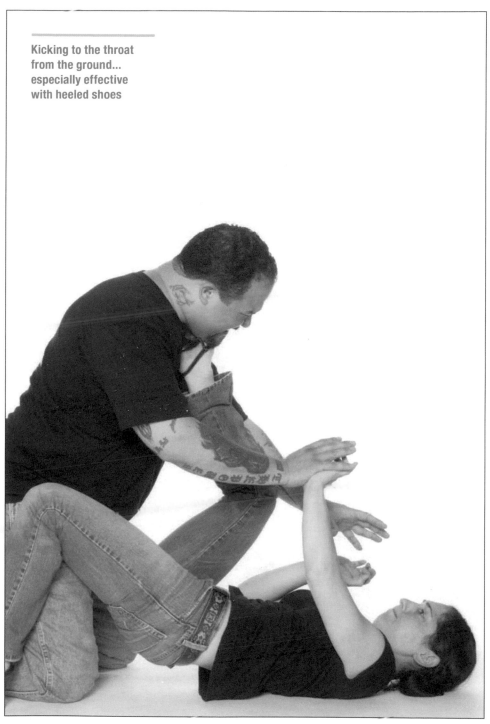

Groin: punches, slapping, chopping, pounding, kicking, knees, biting, squeezing (with crushing intensity), or striking with any defense tool you might have a chance to implement.

If any of these areas are not available, you must target any part of the attacker's body you can reach so that you can deter his attack with resistance, cause pain to change his mind and enable your escape.

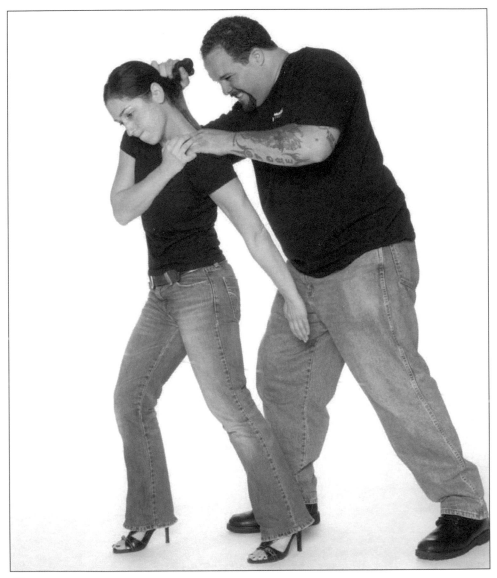

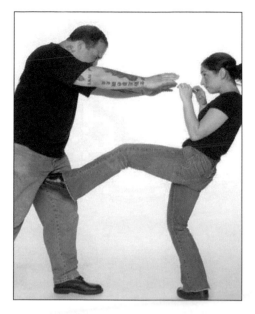
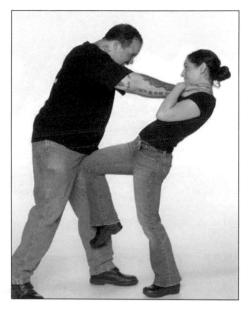

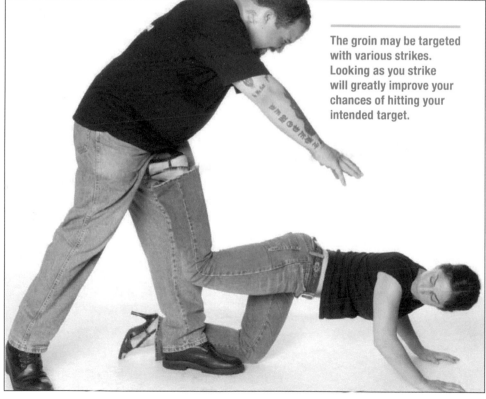

The groin may be targeted with various strikes. Looking as you strike will greatly improve your chances of hitting your intended target.

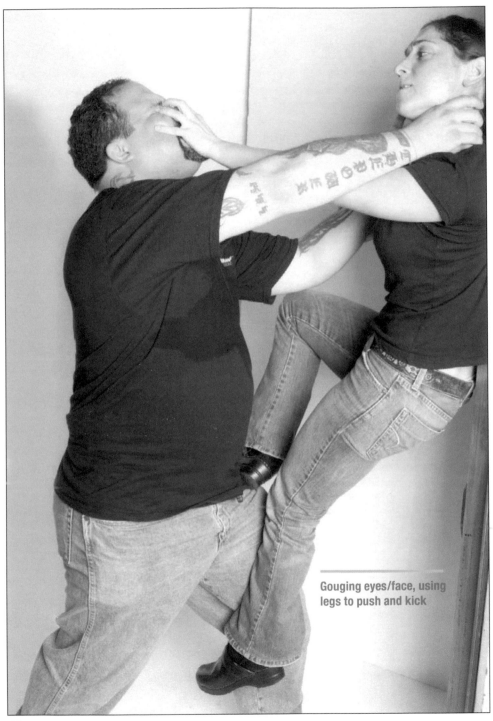

Gouging eyes/face, using legs to push and kick

Situations

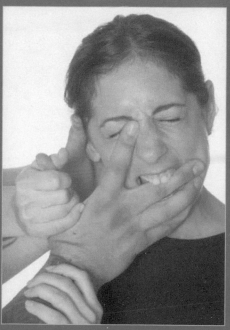

If you think you are **being followed**, stop at the nearest store, deli etc. Explain your situation. Wait a few moments, observe if the person continued on or stopped outside. If possible, call a family member to pick you up and call the police.

If you're unsure whether a person is following you change direction abruptly and see if that person does the same. Let that person know that you are aware of their presence. Show that you're attentive. Try not to panic, slightly increase your pace, and then refer to the first course of action described. Stop into any store or business and call the police. Remember, you can gain attention by blowing a safety whistle at anytime. This will draw the attention that you want and possibly deter a pursuer, because the last thing he wants is attention.

Being attacked/abducted/raped

There are no exceptions, fight for your life. Review all natural body defenses and everyday weapons. Look for opportunities to disable/distract your attacker. An attacker that is trying to remove you from the location has little or no intention of letting you go. If you are completely caught off guard, try to remain calm and pick your moment. If the attacker has a weapon, don't walk with him. Say that you feel terribly sick and can barely stand, abruptly break away and run putting distance and anything you can in between you and the perpetrator. If running isn't possible fall to the ground and begin your defenses, scream, blow your whistle, kick at the attacker's legs and groin, and most importantly, keep your legs and feet in between you and the attacker. If you can't get to your feet and run, your legs and feet are going to be your strongest offensive defense, along with any commotion you can cause. Use any means available to strike the attackers' body. Deceptive tactics can be used to distract your attacker, lead him to believe you're going to comply. Tell him, "I'll do anything you want, don't hurt me, I'm so afraid", remember, you've been caught off guard, so you must turn the tables on your adversary. Try to get your hands close to vital attack areas, his eyes or throat. Maybe close the distance so you can strike his groin or stomp, his foot (instep). If you do nothing, you will most likely be assaulted and or killed.

44

Important note: If being choked, you must, I repeat you must get at least one hand away from your throat. You only have a few moments before you pass out or are left gasping for air. Focus all your attention on getting the hands away from your throat. Snatching at the hands from above and outward to side is your best chance. Trying to muscle the hands will be a waste of precious energy. While freeing the grip on your throat try to knee and kick to groin. If the perpetrator's arms are bent you may be able to strike his face and throat.

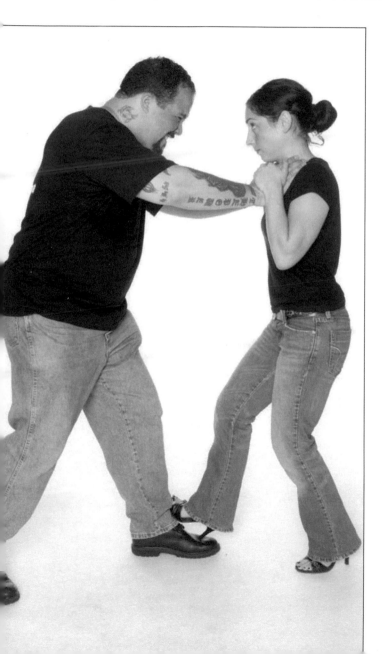

Heel stomp to instep of attacker foot (can scrape down shin)

QUICK OFFENSIVE DEFENSES

Implement these offensive strikes as soon as you can reach the perpetrator/s.

Quick kick to the groin

Quick kick to the shin

Quick poke (single or all fingers) to the eyes

Slap at the eyes, nose or ears with the palm

Punch at the eyes, nose or throat

Chop at the throat (front or side)

Grab and break finger or fingers

Quick bite: to any body part

Attacker Behind You:

Heel kick to the shin, stomp the instep

Slap the groin

Back of your head to the face

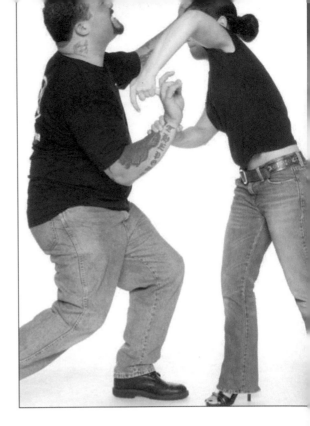

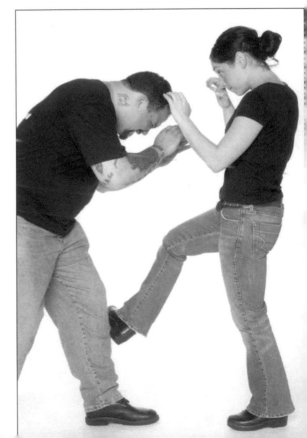

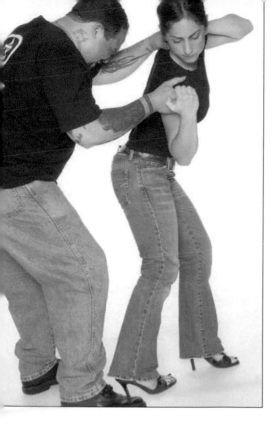

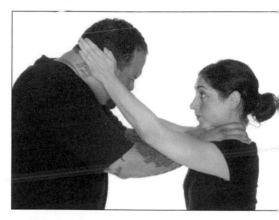

Remember there are no rules!
Whatever, however;
DO SOMETHING AND GET OUT
OF THERE!

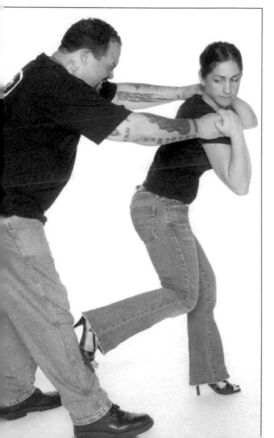

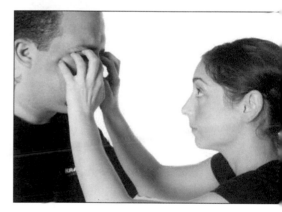

Left page: Finger break
Heel kick and shin scrape
Right page: Heel stomp
to instep
Ear Slaps/Eye gouge
Heel kick to knee

Safety items:

Whistle: provides loud distraction, alerts, saves energy if you're injured and can't keep calling for help, cheap, can be kept readily available, and can be used as a weapon in the hand to scrape or poke sensitive areas.

Small Light: for a couple of dollars there are reliable mini lights that can be an invaluable resource for use during power failures or your car breaks down in the middle of the night or for going down an unlit stairwell.

Small pocket knife: great for cutting a restraint (seat belt) or entanglement, cutting clothing caught in a train or elevator door or for defensive purposes as a **last resort**.

Get used to the operation of these safety items!

Car fire: safety tool, (seatbelt cutter / window hammer / flashlight) all-in-one, available at any major car supplies store. These days most cars come with power windows and door locks. A collision that jams the doors and interrupts electrical power will prevent the window and door operation. In case of fire, you will need to possibly cut the seat belt, break the window and escape to safety. This tool will facilitate all of the above. You can also carry an approved fire extinguisher for assistance with putting out the fire.

Please note; most vehicles made in 2002 and after have installed emergency release latches inside the trunk area. Please familiarize yourself with this feature if it is available in your car. If not, take the time to investigate whether your vehicles trunk can be opened by other means, such as pulling the trunk cable that disengages the latch. The time invested may save your life. The trunk may be an alternate means of escape during a fire or attempted abduction.

Most cars with alarms have a panic feature built into the remote device. This feature sets off the alarm when the button or buttons are held for a few consecutive seconds. This can be a means of alerting the authorities and or people around you that something is wrong.

House fire: tools, flashlight, whistle, fire extinguishers and smoke alarms for each floor, escape ladder kept readily accessible in hall closet. An escape plan that should be reviewed by all house occupants on a regular basis.

Building fire: tools, small light, whistle. Know your escape routes, ask building manager for escape route plan, larger buildings will have them posted near stair wells or elevator banks.

Be Safe!

Remember Be aware Be prepared Escape and Survive!

Written by **Ed Maisonet**

A product of LifeDefenseInc   Contact info: LifeDefense@aol.com

About Ed Maisonet:

I am a Krav Maga Self-Defense Instructor.....a system which was developed for the Israeli Defense Forces and has been expanded for civilian use. I train and teach at John Jay College in Manhattan under the supervision of Master Krav Maga Instructor Rhon Mizrachi, who is a life long practitioner of the art and protégé of Haim Zut, one of the founders of Krav Maga and the highest ranking Krav Maga Instructor alive. I also have my own school located in Staten Island, New York. I served in the United States Navy and participated in Operation Desert Shield and Operation Desert Storm. I've been an armed guard with the responsibilities of protecting people, property and currency deliveries and the transfer of precious metals and stones. I held the position of driver/bodyguard for seven years in Manhattan. With the responsibility of transporting and protecting many high profile clients for one of the largest and influential law firms on the East coast. Planning and practice have been my most valuable assets, which enable me to respond to the unforeseen situations that can arise at any moment

About Leslie Meisel:

She is an actress in New York City and since moving here and working in a bar, felt the necessity for women to learn how to protect themselves in any situation. She has supported this project from day one and stated "she is proud to be part of it". lesliemeisel@yahoo.com

Eddie and Leslie first met while taking Krav Maga Self-Defense at John Jay College. Eddie being one of the biggest in class and Leslie being one of the smallest made this a perfect example why a system of self-defense must depend on technique and strategy, not strength or size.

Contributing Editor: Allison Butterfass: albutterfass@gmail.com

Contributing Editor: Michele Farbman: mfarbman@aol.com

Thank you to my family and friends for believing...
and for all the support!

My name is Ed Maisonet and my goal is to remind everyone of their first and most basic function…Self-Preservation. The need for self/survival-defense awareness and training has somehow been left off of life's basic skills list. No longer can we leave our preventative safety in the hands of others…We must educate ourselves with the basic information available with regard to life threatening situations and the bad guys that may come with them. Too often we look to others to save the day. With some invested time and practice everyone can prepare themselves for those unexpected situations that can change our lives in the blink of an eye.

I'm a Krav Maga Self-Defense Instructor. A system which was developed for the Israeli Defense Forces and has been expanded for civilian use. I train and teach at John Jay College in Manhattan (KravMagaFederation.com), under the supervision of Master Krav Maga Instructor Rhon Mizrachi, who is a life long practitioner of the art and protégé of Haim Zut, the highest ranking Krav Maga Instructor alive. I also have my own school located in Staten Island (LifeDefenseInc.com), New York. I served in the United States Navy and participated in Operation Desert Shield and Operation Desert Storm. I've been an armed guard with the responsibilities of protecting property, currency deliveries and the transfer of precious metals and stones. I held the position of driver/bodyguard for many years in Manhattan. With the responsibility of transporting and protecting many high profile clients for one of the most prestigious law firms on the East coast. Planning and practice have been my most valuable assets, which enable me to respond to the unforeseen situations that can arise at any moment.

The measures described in this guide are not specialized techniques, but basic principles, concepts and movements that everyone can understand and employ.

Made in the USA
Charleston, SC
14 June 2010